Fasting and Cancer

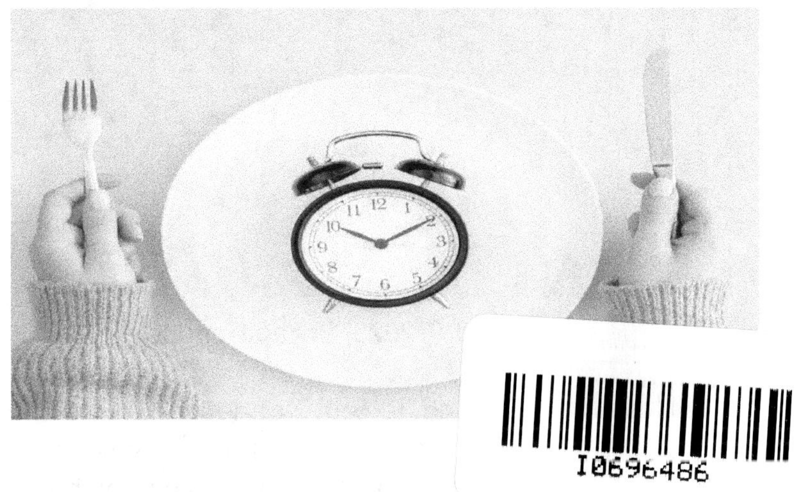

Guide to Healing the Body Through
Fasting and Losing Weight the
Natural Way

ISAAC HENDRICKS

Table of Contents

INTRODUCTION

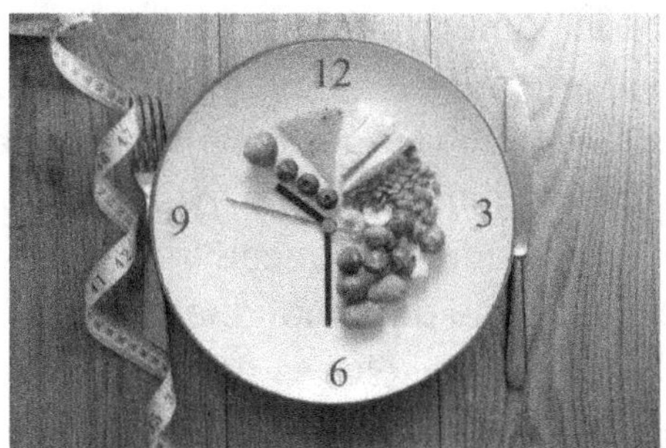

Introduction to Fasting and Cancer

Overview of Fasting

Fasting has gained significant attention in recent years as a potential complementary treatment for cancer. This overview aims to explore the relationship between fasting and cancer, discussing its potential benefits, limitations, and current scientific research.

Fasting is the practice of abstaining from food or specific types of food for an extended period of time. For millennia, it has been done for a variety of reasons, including religious, spiritual, and health grounds. In the context of cancer, fasting is being investigated for its potential to enhance the effectiveness of cancer treatments and reduce side effects.

One of the primary mechanisms through which fasting is believed to impact cancer is by targeting the metabolic pathways that cancer cells rely on for their growth and survival. Fasting can promote a metabolic state known as ketosis, where the body shifts from using glucose as its main fuel source to utilising ketone bodies produced from stored fat. Cancer cells, on the other hand, are thought to be less efficient in using ketones as an energy source, which may result in their inhibition or selective killing.

Additionally, fasting has been found to increase the levels of certain hormones and molecules in the body, such as insulin-like growth factor 1 (IGF-1) and adiponectin, which may have anti-cancer effects. Moreover, fasting has been found to stimulate autophagy, a natural cellular process that involves the recycling and elimination of damaged or dysfunctional molecules and organelles, which could help in stopping or halting the progression of cancer.

While there is a growing body of preclinical and clinical evidence suggesting that fasting may have beneficial effects in cancer, it is important to note that most of the research conducted so far has been in animal models or small-scale human studies. Therefore, the results should be interpreted with caution, and more large-scale, controlled trials are needed to establish the safety and efficacy of fasting as a therapeutic approach for cancer.

It is also crucial to highlight that fasting alone is not a substitute for conventional cancer treatments such as surgery, chemotherapy, or radiation therapy. Instead, fasting is being investigated as a complementary strategy that can potentially enhance the effectiveness of these treatments and reduce their side effects. Therefore, any decision regarding fasting as a part of cancer treatment should be made in consultation with healthcare professionals.

In conclusion, fasting is an emerging area of research in the field of cancer treatment and prevention. While its potential benefits, such as metabolic modulation and stimulation of autophagy, are promising, more rigorous studies are needed to validate its efficacy and safety. Clinicians and researchers are actively exploring fasting as a potential complementary approach to improve cancer treatment outcomes, but it is essential to approach this field with scientific rigour and caution.

Understanding Cancer

Cancer is a complicated and complex disease that affects millions of individuals worldwide. It is characterised by the uncontrolled growth and division of abnormal cells in the body, leading to the formation of tumours. Cancer can occur in any part of the body and can have life-changing consequences for both patients and their families. However, understanding the underlying causes, risk factors, and treatment options is crucial in developing effective prevention strategies and improving patient outcomes. In this article, we will explore the fundamental aspects of cancer, shedding light on the various dimensions of this disease.

What is Cancer?

Cancer is a term used to describe a group of diseases characterised by the uncontrolled growth and spread of abnormal cells. Normally, cells in the body grow, divide, and then die in an orderly fashion. However, in cancer, this process goes awry. The abnormal cells continue to divide and accumulate, forming a mass called a tumour. Tumours are classified as either malignant (cancerous) or benign (non-cancerous). Malignant tumours have the ability to invade and infiltrate nearby tissues and organs, while benign tumors remain localised and do not spread.

Causes and Risk Factors:

While the exact cause of cancer is often unknown, there are several risk factors associated with its development. Genetic mutations, environmental factors, lifestyle choices, and certain infections can all contribute to the onset of cancer. Genetic mutations can be inherited through generations or acquired throughout one's lifetime, and they play a critical role in the development of certain types of cancer. Environmental factors such as exposure to carcinogens, radiation, and certain chemicals can also increase the risk of developing cancer. Lifestyle choices, such as tobacco and alcohol consumption, poor diet, obesity, and lack of physical activity, can significantly contribute to certain types of cancer. Additionally, certain viral and bacterial infections, such as human papillomavirus (HPV) and hepatitis B and C viruses, are known to cause specific types of cancer.

Types of Cancer:

There are more than 100 types of cancer, each with its own distinct characteristics and behaviours. Some common types include breast cancer, lung cancer, prostate cancer, colorectal cancer, and skin cancer. The type of cancer determines the treatment approach and prognosis for each individual. While advances in research have led to improved diagnostic methods and targeted therapies for specific cancers, many challenges still exist in effectively treating certain types of cancer.

Diagnosis and Treatment:

Early detection and diagnosis are critical for successful cancer treatment. Various screening tests, imaging techniques, and biopsies are used to confirm the presence of cancer, determine its stage, and plan the appropriate treatment. Treatment options for cancer vary depending on the type, stage, and overall health of the patient. Common treatment modalities include surgery, radiation therapy, chemotherapy, immunotherapy, targeted therapy, and hormone therapy. Additionally, there are ongoing advancements in precision medicine and personalised therapies that aim to tailor treatment options to individual patients based on their genetic makeup.

Prevention and Support:

Prevention and risk reduction strategies, such as regular exercise, healthy eating, avoiding tobacco and excessive alcohol use, and protecting oneself from exposure to harmful environmental factors, are crucial in reducing the incidence of cancer. Additionally, vaccinations against certain infections can also prevent the development of specific cancers. For those currently battling cancer, support systems, including emotional, psychological, and financial support, are essential in navigating the challenges associated with diagnosis and treatment. Various organisations and communities provide resources and services to aid and empower cancer patients and their families.

Conclusion:

Understanding cancer is an ongoing and dynamic process, with constant advancements in research and medical technology. While cancer remains a formidable challenge, progress is being made in various aspects of cancer prevention, diagnosis, and treatment. Through education and awareness, individuals can make informed decisions about their health and adopt strategies to reduce their risk of developing cancer. Continued research and collaboration among researchers, healthcare professionals, and policymakers hold the key to further improving cancer outcomes and eventually finding a cure.

Link between Fasting and Cancer

There is an emerging body of research suggesting a link between fasting and cancer prevention, treatment, and even improved outcomes for cancer patients. Fasting, defined as voluntarily abstaining from food and sometimes fluids for a certain period of time, has been practised for centuries due to religious, cultural, or health reasons. Over the years, scientists have discovered that fasting triggers various physiological changes in the body that can positively impact cancer.

One of the key mechanisms by which fasting may affect cancer is through the regulation of insulin and insulin-like growth factor 1 (IGF-1) levels. Both insulin and IGF-1 are growth factors that stimulate the growth and proliferation of cells, including cancer cells. High insulin and IGF-1 levels have been linked to an increased risk of developing certain types of cancer, such as breast, colorectal, and prostate cancer.

By fasting, individuals can lower their insulin and IGF-1 levels, which in turn may inhibit the growth of cancer cells and reduce the risk of tumour formation. Fasting has also been found to improve the effectiveness of chemotherapy drugs, as cancer cells rely heavily on glucose as an energy source, and fasting can deplete glucose levels in the body. This deprivation of glucose can make cancer cells more vulnerable and susceptible to the cytotoxic effects of chemotherapy drugs.

Additionally, fasting has been shown to activate a cellular self-defence mechanism called autophagy. Autophagy is a process in which damaged or dysfunctional cells are broken down and recycled, thus promoting cellular renewal and removing potential cancerous cells. It is believed that fasting-induced autophagy may help prevent the development and progression of cancer by eliminating damaged DNA and other cellular components that could lead to malignant transformation.

Furthermore, fasting has been shown to increase the production of ketone bodies, which are used as an alternative fuel source when glucose is limited. Some studies suggest that cancer cells have a reduced ability to use ketones for energy compared to healthy cells. This metabolic difference between cancer cells and normal cells could potentially be exploited through fasting or ketogenic diets to starve cancer cells while protecting healthy cells.

It is important to note that while there is growing evidence supporting the potential benefits of fasting in cancer prevention and treatment, more research is needed to fully understand the underlying mechanisms and determine the optimal fasting protocols for specific cancer types and stages. Additionally, fasting may not be suitable for everyone, especially those with certain medical conditions or nutritional deficiencies. Therefore, it is essential to consult with a healthcare professional before considering any fasting regimen for cancer-related purposes.

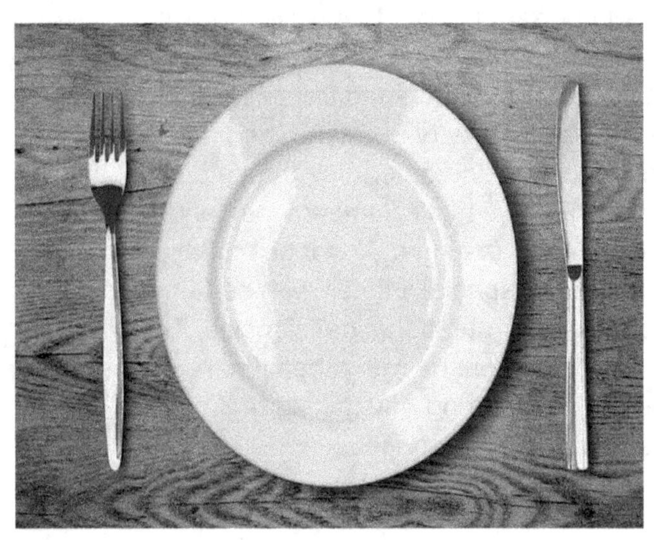

CHAPTER ONE

Fasting and Cancer: Mechanisms and Benefits

Autophagy and Cancer Cells

Autophagy is a cellular process that plays a crucial role in the maintenance of cellular homeostasis. It involves the degradation and recycling of damaged organelles, misfolded proteins, and intracellular pathogens. Autophagy ensures the elimination of dysfunctional components and the availability of essential nutrients during times of stress, such as nutrient deprivation, hypoxia, or cellular damage.

Cancer cells are characterised by uncontrolled proliferation and the ability to evade cell death mechanisms. Autophagy can have both tumour-promoting and tumour-suppressing effects, depending on the context and stage of cancer development. Here, we will discuss the complex relationship between autophagy and cancer cells.

In the early stages of cancer development, autophagy acts as a tumour suppressor mechanism. It helps to maintain genomic stability by removing damaged organelles and preventing the accumulation of protein aggregates and toxic metabolites. Autophagy also plays a critical role in the prevention of inflammation and cell death that could potentially promote tumour initiation or progression.

However, as cancer progresses, the relationship between autophagy and cancer cells becomes more complicated. In established tumours, cancer cells often exploit autophagy as a survival mechanism. Tumour cells can activate autophagy to overcome nutrient and oxygen deprivation, which is a common feature of the tumour microenvironment. By recycling intracellular components, cancer cells can ensure their survival under adverse conditions, facilitating tumour growth and resistance to therapy.

Furthermore, autophagy can also be induced in response to cancer therapies such as radiation or chemotherapy. This can be either beneficial or detrimental to the outcome of the treatment, depending on the specific circumstances. On one hand, autophagy can help cancer cells to survive the stress induced by therapy, leading to treatment resistance. On the other hand, excessive autophagy can result in cellular self-destruction, ultimately promoting cell death and tumour regression.

Given the dual role of autophagy in cancer, it has become an attractive target for cancer therapy. Several drugs that modulate autophagy have been developed and tested in preclinical and clinical studies. These drugs aim to either inhibit autophagy to sensitise cancer cells to therapy or induce autophagy to trigger cell death in cancer cells.

In conclusion, autophagy is a complex process that plays a significant role in cancer cells. While it acts as a tumour suppressor in the early stages of cancer development, it can become a survival mechanism in established tumours. Understanding the intricate relationship between autophagy and cancer cells is crucial for the development of effective cancer therapies. Further research in this area will provide insights into exploiting autophagy for therapeutic purposes, ultimately improving the treatment outcomes for cancer patients.

Impact of Fasting on Tumour Growth

Fasting is defined as a voluntary abstinence from food and/or drink for a particular period of time. It has been practised for religious, spiritual, and health reasons for centuries. Recent research has revealed that fasting can have a profound impact on various aspects of health, including tumour growth.

Tumours are abnormal cell masses that grow uncontrollably and can be either benign or malignant. Cancerous tumours, in particular, can be highly invasive and spread to other parts of the body, causing significant morbidity and mortality. Understanding the potential effects of fasting on tumour growth is crucial in developing new treatment strategies for cancer patients.

During fasting, the body enters a state of energy conservation due to the lack of external energy sources. This state triggers multiple metabolic adaptations that can influence tumour development. One of the main adaptations is the activation of the cellular process known as autophagy. Autophagy is a natural mechanism in which cells break down and recycle damaged proteins and organelles to generate energy. This process has been shown to inhibit tumour growth and promote tumour cell death in various types of cancer.

Additionally, fasting can limit the availability of glucose, which is the primary fuel source for cancer cells. Cancer cells have a high demand for glucose to support their rapid growth and division. By depriving tumour cells of glucose, fasting can induce a metabolic stress that impairs their survival and proliferation. This metabolic stress can also sensitise tumours to standard cancer therapies, such as chemotherapy and radiation therapy, enhancing their effectiveness.

Furthermore, fasting can modulate the immune system and enhance anti-tumor immune responses. Studies have demonstrated that fasting can stimulate the production of certain immune cells, such as natural killer cells and T cells, which are critical in recognizing and eliminating cancer cells. Fasting can also reduce inflammation in the body, which is often associated with tumour growth and progression.

Although the impact of fasting on tumour growth has been primarily studied in preclinical models and limited clinical trials, the results are promising. Animal studies have shown that fasting can significantly delay tumour progression and improve survival rates. In human trials, fasting has demonstrated potential as an adjuvant therapy to enhance the efficacy of cancer treatments and reduce treatment-related side effects.

It is crucial to remember, however, that fasting is not a treatment for cancer. It should be considered as a complementary approach to conventional cancer treatments, and its implementation should be carefully monitored and tailored to each individual's specific condition and needs.

In conclusion, fasting has emerged as a potentially impactful strategy for inhibiting tumour growth. By promoting autophagy, restricting glucose availability, and modulating the immune system, fasting can exert multiple effects on cancer cells, enhancing their vulnerability and improving treatment outcomes. Further research is needed to better understand the mechanisms underlying the impact of fasting on tumour growth and to develop safe and effective fasting protocols for cancer patients.

Effects of Fasting on Cancer Treatment and Chemotherapy

Several studies have investigated the effects of fasting on cancer treatment and chemotherapy, and the results have been promising. Here are some of the most important findings:

1. Enhanced efficacy of chemotherapy: Fasting has been shown to enhance the efficacy of chemotherapy drugs by making cancer cells more susceptible to the toxic effects of these drugs. Fasting has been found to promote the selective death of tumour cells while leaving healthy cells relatively unharmed.

2. Reduced side effects: Chemotherapy often causes various side effects, including nausea, vomiting, and fatigue. Fasting has been suggested to mitigate these side effects by improving the overall tolerance and response to chemotherapy drugs. Fasting has been found to increase the body's resistance to stress and reduce the toxic impact of chemotherapy on healthy tissues.

3. Reduced tumour growth and progression: Fasting has been shown to inhibit the growth and progression of tumours by reducing the availability

of nutrients that cancer cells need to proliferate. Fasting triggers several signalling pathways in the body that can suppress tumour growth and metastasis.

4. Enhanced immune system function: Fasting has been found to enhance the function of the immune system, which plays a crucial role in fighting cancer. It stimulates the production of immune cells and improves their ability to recognize and eliminate cancer cells.

5. Protection of healthy cells: Fasting has been shown to protect healthy cells from the toxic effects of chemotherapy, thus reducing potential damage to healthy tissues. This protection is believed to be mediated by the activation of various cellular repair mechanisms and increased production of protective molecules.

It is important to note that fasting should be approached with caution and under medical supervision, especially for cancer patients undergoing treatment. The timing, duration, and specific protocols of fasting may vary depending on individual health conditions and treatment plans.

In conclusion, fasting has demonstrated several beneficial effects on cancer treatment and chemotherapy. It can enhance the effectiveness of chemotherapy, reduce side effects, inhibit tumour growth, boost immune system function, and protect healthy cells. However, further research is still needed to determine the optimal fasting protocols and their integration with standard cancer treatment strategies. Therefore, it is recommended that individuals consult with their healthcare providers before incorporating fasting into their cancer treatment regimen.

Potential Benefits of Fasting in Cancer Prevention

Fasting has been a topic of interest in recent years for its potential benefits in cancer prevention. While research in this area is still ongoing, there is emerging evidence suggesting that fasting may help in reducing the risk of various types of cancer. Here are some potential benefits of fasting in cancer prevention:

1. Enhanced immune response: Fasting has been found to stimulate autophagy, a cellular recycling process that removes damaged cells and promotes the regeneration of healthy cells. This can help strengthen the immune system and reduce the risk of cancer development.

2. Reduced inflammation: Prolonged fasting has been shown to decrease inflammation in the body. Chronic inflammation is associated with an increased risk of cancer, so by reducing inflammation, fasting may help lower the likelihood of cancer occurrence.

3. Metabolic effects: Fasting can have various metabolic effects such as improved insulin sensitivity, decreased insulin-like growth factor 1 (IGF-1) levels, and increased ketone production. These changes in the body's metabolism may help create an unfavourable environment for cancer cells to grow and proliferate.

4. Protection of healthy cells: Research suggests that fasting may selectively protect healthy cells while making cancer cells more vulnerable to treatments like chemotherapy and radiation. By creating a metabolic state that favours healthy cells, fasting may help limit the side effects of cancer treatments.

5. Delayed tumour growth: Animal studies have shown that intermittent fasting can lead to delayed tumour growth and reduced cancer cell proliferation. While human studies are still limited, the findings suggest that fasting has the potential to slow down the progression of cancer.

It's important to note that fasting should always be approached with caution, especially for individuals undergoing cancer treatments or with underlying health conditions. Consulting with a healthcare professional, particularly an oncologist or registered dietitian, is crucial in determining whether fasting is safe and appropriate for each individual's specific situation.

In conclusion, while more research is needed to fully understand the effects of fasting on cancer prevention, the potential benefits are promising. Fasting may positively impact the immune system, reduce inflammation, alter metabolism, protect healthy cells, and potentially slow down tumour growth. However, it is always advisable to seek professional guidance and individualise the approach based on one's unique circumstances.

CHAPTER TWO

Different Approaches to Fasting for Cancer Patients

Intermittent Fasting

Intermittent fasting is a dietary approach that has gained significant attention in recent years due to its potential health benefits. Many cancer patients wonder if this approach could benefit them during their treatment journey. In this article, we will explore the concept of intermittent fasting and its potential impact on cancer patients.

Intermittent fasting entails alternate intervals of fasting and eating. The most common method is the 16/8 regimen, where people fast for 16 hours and then eat during an 8-hour window. Other variations include alternate-day fasting or 24-hour fasting once or twice a week.

Research on intermittent fasting in cancer patients is still limited, but there are some promising findings. Some studies conducted on animals have shown that intermittent fasting can help slow down the growth of cancer cells and enhance the effectiveness of chemotherapy drugs. Additionally, fasting has been found to potentially reduce the side effects of chemotherapy, such as fatigue and nausea, and improve overall well-being during treatment.

One of the proposed mechanisms behind the benefits of intermittent fasting in cancer patients is the activation of autophagy. Autophagy is a process where damaged or dysfunctional cells are broken down and recycled. By stimulating autophagy through fasting, it is believed that cancer cells could be targeted and destroyed more effectively.

Moreover, intermittent fasting has been associated with improvements in metabolic health and insulin sensitivity. Cancer patients undergoing treatment often experience weight gain or metabolic dysregulation, putting them at a higher risk of diabetes and other chronic diseases. Intermittent fasting may help regulate blood sugar levels and promote weight loss, which could aid in symptom management and recovery.

However, it is important to note that intermittent fasting may not be suitable for all cancer patients. The impact of fasting could vary depending on the type and stage of cancer, as well as the individual's overall health status. Therefore, it is crucial for cancer patients to consult with their healthcare team before implementing any dietary changes, including intermittent fasting.

Additionally, cancer patients should be cautious about maintaining adequate nutrition during their treatment. Fasting can restrict calorie intake, which may lead to nutrient deficiencies if not carefully planned. Therefore, it is essential for patients to work closely with a registered dietitian or nutritionist to ensure their nutritional needs are met while incorporating intermittent fasting.

In conclusion, intermittent fasting shows potential as a complementary approach for cancer patients. It may help inhibit cancer cell growth, enhance the effectiveness of chemotherapy, and improve overall well-being. However, it is essential for patients to consult with their healthcare team and obtain individualised guidance on incorporating intermittent fasting into their treatment plan.

Prolonged Fasting

Prolonged fasting, also known as extended fasting, is a practice that involves abstaining from food for an extended period of time. While it has gained popularity as a method for weight loss and overall health improvement, there is growing interest in its potential benefits for cancer patients. This concept of fasting has gained attention due to its ability to possibly enhance the effectiveness of cancer treatments while reducing the side effects.

Cancer is a complex disease that requires multiple treatment modalities, including surgery, chemotherapy, radiation therapy, and targeted therapies. While these treatments have improved over the years, they often come with side effects that can be debilitating for patients. Prolonged fasting has been suggested as a complementary approach to conventional cancer treatment, with the potential to improve both its efficacy and tolerance.

Studies on animals have shown promising results regarding the impact of fasting on cancer cells. Research suggests that prolonged fasting can induce metabolic changes in cancer cells, leading to increased sensitiveness to chemotherapy and radiation therapy. Fasting may also stimulate the immune system, contributing to the body's ability to control and eliminate cancer cells. Furthermore, it has been observed that fasting can provide a protective effect on healthy cells, making them more resilient to the toxic effects of cancer treatments.

Apart from enhancing traditional cancer treatments, prolonged fasting has also shown potential for reducing side effects. It has been reported that fasting can decrease the severity and occurrence of common chemotherapy side effects such as nausea, vomiting, and fatigue. This could greatly improve the quality of life for cancer patients undergoing treatment and provide them with a better overall experience.

However, it is important to note that the research on prolonged fasting for cancer patients is still in its early stages and primarily based on animal models and small human studies. The effects of fasting may vary depending on various factors, including cancer type, treatment plan, and the overall health of the patient. Therefore, it is crucial for cancer patients to consult their healthcare provider before considering prolonged fasting as part of their treatment strategy.

In conclusion, prolonged fasting holds promise as a complementary approach for cancer patients. Its potential to enhance the efficacy of cancer treatments while minimising side effects makes it an intriguing area of research. However, more comprehensive studies are needed to establish the optimal fasting protocols, safety guidelines, and long-term effects on cancer outcomes. It is essential for patients to discuss these options with their medical team to determine the suitability and potential benefits of prolonged fasting in their individual cases.

Caloric Restriction Mimicking Diets (CRMD)

Caloric Restriction Mimicking Diets (CRMD) have gained attention in recent years for their potential benefits in various health conditions, including cancer. These diets aim to replicate the physiological effects of caloric restriction, which is the practice of reducing calorie intake without causing malnutrition. While research is ongoing, there is evidence to suggest that CRMD may have positive implications for cancer patients. It's important to note that any dietary changes for cancer patients should be discussed with healthcare professionals to ensure they align with the individual's overall treatment plan.

Understanding Caloric Restriction Mimicking Diets (CRMD) for Cancer Patients:

Definition of CRMD:

- CRMD involves cycles of reduced calorie intake, typically lasting for a short duration (a few days), followed by a return to normal calorie consumption. This cycle is intended to mimic the effects of continuous caloric restriction.

Physiological Effects:

- Research suggests that CRMD may induce metabolic changes associated with caloric restriction, such as increased autophagy and improved cellular repair mechanisms. These processes could potentially affect cancer cells.

Influence on Cancer Cells:

- Some preclinical studies have indicated that caloric restriction may have anti-cancer effects by inhibiting the growth and progression of tumours. CRMD, by extension, may exert similar effects due to the simulated metabolic conditions.

Enhanced Sensitivity to Treatment:

- CRMD might enhance the sensitivity of cancer cells to conventional cancer treatments like chemotherapy and radiation. This is an area of ongoing research, and more studies are needed to establish the extent of its effectiveness.

Reduction of Side Effects:

- Caloric restriction, if managed appropriately, may potentially reduce the side effects of cancer treatments. Some evidence suggests that it could mitigate the toxic effects of certain therapies on healthy cells.

Caution and Individualization:

- CRMD may not be suitable for all cancer patients, and its feasibility depends on factors such as the type and stage of cancer, overall health, and individual response. Consulting with healthcare providers, including oncologists and dietitians, is crucial.

Nutrient-Rich Diet:

- While restricting calories, it's vital to ensure that the patient receives essential nutrients. A well-balanced, nutrient-dense diet is crucial to support the body's nutritional needs during and after CRMD cycles.

Patient Monitoring:

- Regular medical supervision and monitoring are essential for cancer patients following CRMD.

Changes in weight, nutritional status, and overall health should be closely tracked to adjust the dietary plan as needed.

Integration with Standard Treatment:
   - CRMD should not be considered a standalone treatment for cancer. It is crucial to integrate it into the overall treatment plan, working in conjunction with established therapies recommended by healthcare professionals.

In conclusion, while the potential benefits of Caloric Restriction Mimicking Diets for cancer patients are intriguing, more research is needed to establish their efficacy and safety. Any dietary changes for cancer patients should be made in consultation with healthcare providers to ensure they align with the individual's specific condition and treatment plan.

Fasting-Mimicking Diet (FMD)

The Fasting-Mimicking Diet (FMD) is a dietary approach that aims to replicate some of the benefits of traditional fasting while still allowing for the consumption of certain foods. The concept behind FMD is to provide the body with a reduced calorie and nutrient intake, which may promote cellular regeneration, enhance stress resistance, and have potential benefits for overall health.

As of my last knowledge update in January 2022, there was some research interest in exploring the potential application of fasting or fasting-mimicking diets in cancer treatment. However, it's essential to note that the field of nutrition and its relationship to cancer is complex, and scientific understanding may evolve over time.

Here are some points to consider regarding FMD for cancer patients:

Preclinical Studies:
Some preclinical studies (studies conducted in animals or cells) have suggested that fasting or FMD may have anti-cancer effects. These effects are thought to be related to changes in metabolic pathways, reduced inflammation, and increased stress resistance in normal cells compared to cancer cells.

Clinical Research:
Clinical trials investigating the use of fasting or FMD in cancer patients were ongoing or in the early stages as of my last update. The goal of these trials is to assess the safety and potential efficacy of incorporating fasting or FMD into cancer treatment protocols.

Individualised Approach:
Cancer is a heterogeneous disease, meaning it can vary significantly from person to person. The response to dietary interventions, including FMD, may also vary among individuals. It's crucial for any dietary approach, especially in the context of

cancer treatment, to be personalised based on the patient's specific circumstances.

Medical Supervision:
If a cancer patient is considering trying an FMD or any other dietary intervention, it's crucial to do so under the supervision of healthcare professionals, including oncologists and registered dietitians. Cancer treatment plans are complex, and dietary changes should be integrated into the overall care plan in a way that supports the patient's health and well-being.

Potential Risks:
Fasting or drastic changes in diet may pose risks, especially for individuals undergoing cancer treatment. Malnutrition and unintended weight loss can be concerns. Therefore, any dietary changes should be carefully monitored to ensure they do not compromise the patient's nutritional status.

It's important to consult with healthcare professionals who are familiar with the individual's medical history and treatment plan before considering any dietary changes, including FMD, during cancer treatment. Additionally, given that research evolves, it's recommended to check for the latest scientific literature or consult with healthcare providers for the most up-to-date information on this topic.

CHAPTER THREE

Fasting Protocols for Cancer Patients

Safety Considerations and Medical Supervision

Safety considerations and medical supervision are crucial aspects of the care and treatment of cancer patients. Cancer is a complex disease that often requires a multidisciplinary approach, involving various medical professionals to ensure the well-being of the patient. Here are some key points regarding safety considerations and medical supervision for cancer patients:

Safety Considerations:

1. **Infection Control:**
   - Cancer patients, especially those undergoing chemotherapy, may have compromised immune systems. Strict infection control measures should be in place to minimise the risk of infections.
   - Regular handwashing, proper sanitation, and restriction of visitors with illnesses are essential precautions.

2. Chemotherapy Safety:

- Chemotherapy drugs are potent and can have significant side effects. Safety protocols must be followed when administering these drugs to minimise the risk of adverse reactions.

- Adequate training for healthcare professionals involved in chemotherapy administration is crucial to ensure proper handling and disposal of these medications.

3. Fall Prevention:

- Some cancer treatments and medications can cause weakness or imbalance. Fall prevention measures, such as non-slip flooring, handrails, and assistance with mobility, should be implemented.

4. Nutritional Support:

- Malnutrition is common among cancer patients due to the disease itself and the side effects of treatments. Nutritional support and monitoring are essential to maintain the patient's strength and immune function.

5. Pain Management:

- Adequate pain management is crucial for the comfort and well-being of cancer patients. Regular assessment and adjustment of pain medications should be carried out under the supervision of healthcare professionals.

1. Ongoing Monitoring:
- Regular medical check-ups and monitoring of vital signs are essential to track the patient's overall health and detect any potential complications early.

2. Individualised Treatment Plans:
- Each cancer patient is unique, and treatment plans should be tailored to their specific needs and health status. Regular adjustments to the treatment plan may be necessary based on the patient's response.

3. Psychosocial Support:
- Cancer patients frequently face emotional and psychological difficulties. Medical supervision should include access to psychosocial support services, such as counselling and support groups.

4. Coordination of Care:
- Collaboration among healthcare professionals involved in the patient's care is crucial. This includes oncologists, nurses, nutritionists, and other specialists working together to provide comprehensive care.

5. Communication with Patients:
- Open and honest communication between healthcare providers and cancer patients is essential. Patients should be informed about their

treatment plans, potential side effects, and what to expect throughout the course of their care.

In conclusion, safety considerations and medical supervision are integral to the comprehensive care of cancer patients. A holistic approach, addressing not only the disease but also the individual needs and challenges of each patient, is essential for optimal outcomes and improved quality of life.

Choosing the Right Fasting Protocol

Fasting has gained attention as a potential complementary approach to cancer treatment, with some studies suggesting that it may enhance the effectiveness of conventional therapies and reduce side effects. However, choosing the right fasting protocol for cancer patients requires careful consideration and consultation with healthcare professionals. Consider the following factors:

1. Individualised Approach:

- Every cancer patient is unique, and there is no one-size-fits-all fasting protocol. Factors such as the type and stage of cancer, overall health, age, and nutritional status should be taken into account.
- Consultation with an oncologist or a healthcare team is crucial to assess the patient's specific situation and determine if fasting is a safe and appropriate option.

2. Types of Fasting:

- Intermittent Fasting: This involves cycles of eating and fasting. The 16/8 approach (16 hours of fasting and an 8-hour eating window) and alternate-day fasting are two popular methods.

- Water Fasting: This typically involves consuming only water for a specified period. Extended water fasting should be supervised by healthcare professionals due to the risk of dehydration and nutrient deficiencies.
- Caloric Restriction: This involves reducing overall calorie intake, potentially slowing down cancer growth. However, maintaining proper nutrition is crucial.

3. Timing in Conjunction with Treatment:

- Fasting around the time of chemotherapy or radiation therapy may help enhance the effectiveness of these treatments, as some studies suggest that fasting may sensitise cancer cells to treatment while protecting normal cells.
- However, the timing of fasting concerning treatment is critical, and coordination with the oncology team is essential to avoid interference with the therapeutic process.

4. Monitoring and Safety:

- Fasting can lead to nutritional deficiencies and other side effects. Regular monitoring of the patient's health, including blood tests and vital signs, is essential.
- Patients should be closely supervised during fasting, and healthcare providers should be informed of any adverse effects promptly.

5. Patient Preferences and Compliance:

- Consideration should be given to the patient's ability to adhere to a fasting protocol. Some individuals may find certain methods more manageable than others.
- Patient preferences and comfort with fasting should be taken into account to ensure compliance with the chosen protocol.

6. Comprehensive Care:

- Fasting should not be viewed as a standalone treatment but as part of a comprehensive care plan. It is essential to continue conventional cancer treatments and supportive care in conjunction with fasting.

In conclusion, while there is emerging evidence supporting the potential benefits of fasting in cancer care, it is crucial to approach it with caution and under the guidance of healthcare professionals.

Fasting should be tailored to individual patient needs, with careful consideration of the type and stage of cancer, overall health, and treatment plan. Always consult with a healthcare team before initiating any fasting protocol for cancer patients.

Adapting Fasting Protocols based on Cancer Type and Stage

Fasting has emerged as a potential adjunct to conventional cancer therapies, with research suggesting its ability to enhance treatment outcomes and reduce side effects. However, the effectiveness of fasting protocols may vary depending on the type and stage of cancer. Tailoring fasting strategies to individual cancer characteristics is crucial for optimising therapeutic benefits and ensuring patient safety.

Understanding Fasting Protocols:

Fasting protocols typically involve cycles of abstaining from food for specific periods. These can include intermittent fasting, where eating is restricted to certain time windows, or more extended fasts lasting several days. The rationale behind fasting in cancer treatment lies in its ability to create a hostile environment for cancer cells while potentially enhancing the body's response to treatment.

1. Solid Tumour Cancers:

   - Fasting may support conventional therapies like chemotherapy and radiation for solid tumours.

   - Extended fasts might be considered for certain solid tumours, with careful monitoring to prevent malnutrition.

2. Haematological Cancers:

   - Intermittent fasting may be beneficial for haematological cancers, as it can potentially enhance the effects of chemotherapy and immunotherapy.

   - Close collaboration with haematologists is crucial to ensure that fasting does not compromise blood counts.

3. Hormone-Driven Cancers:

   - Hormone-driven cancers like breast or prostate cancer may require specific fasting approaches, considering the impact of hormonal changes on cancer progression.

   - Fasting mimicking diets, which provide essential nutrients while mimicking the effects of fasting, might be explored.

Adapting to Cancer Stages:

1. Early-Stage Cancer:

   - Fasting could enhance the effectiveness of localised treatments such as surgery or radiation.

- Short-term fasting before treatment might help sensitise cancer cells to therapy.

2. Advanced-Stage Cancer:

- Short-term fasting may still be beneficial, but extended fasts might require careful consideration due to potential nutritional risks.

- Fasting in conjunction with targeted therapies or immunotherapies may offer a complementary approach.

Considerations and Challenges:

1. Nutritional Support:

- Individualised nutritional plans are essential to prevent malnutrition during fasting.

- Consultation with a nutritionist or dietitian is crucial to address specific dietary needs.

2. Monitoring and Safety:

- Regular medical supervision is necessary to monitor patients for potential side effects and ensure the fasting protocol is well-tolerated.

- Fasting should be adjusted or discontinued if adverse effects arise.

3. Patient Preferences and Compliance:

- The patient's willingness and ability to adhere to fasting protocols should be considered.

- Open communication between patients, oncologists, and nutritionists can enhance compliance and address concerns.

Conclusion:

Adapting fasting protocols based on cancer type and stage represents a promising avenue for personalised cancer care. While research in this field is ongoing, collaboration between oncologists, nutritionists, and patients is crucial for developing safe and effective fasting strategies as part of an integrative approach to cancer treatment. As our understanding of the complex interplay between fasting and cancer continues to grow, personalised fasting protocols may become a valuable tool in the comprehensive management of cancer.

CHAPTER FOUR

Combining Fasting with Conventional Cancer
Treatments

Fasting and Radiation Therapy

Fasting and radiation therapy are two distinct approaches used in cancer treatment, each with its own benefits and considerations. Although fasting has shown potential in enhancing the efficacy of cancer therapy, including radiation therapy, it is essential to approach this topic with caution and consult healthcare professionals before embarking on any fasting regimen during cancer treatment.

Fasting is the voluntary restriction of food intake for a set period. It has long been practised in various religious and cultural traditions, but recent scientific research has revealed its potential impact on cancer treatment as well. Studies in animal models and some early human trials have suggested that fasting may improve the effectiveness of radiation therapy in cancer patients.

One of the key mechanisms behind this possible synergy is the concept of differential stress resistance. Fasting induces a mild metabolic stress response in healthy cells, causing them to adapt and become more resistant to subsequent stressors, such as radiation. In contrast, cancer cells have disrupted metabolism and impaired stress response pathways, making them more vulnerable to radiation-induced damage. This "differential stress resistance" hypothesis suggests that fasting may selectively sensitise cancer cells to radiation while protecting healthy cells.

Moreover, fasting has been found to reduce the levels of insulin-like growth factor 1 (IGF-1) and glucose, both of which play a crucial role in cancer growth and proliferation. By lowering these factors, fasting may create an unfavourable environment for tumour growth and potentially enhance the effectiveness of radiation therapy.

However, it is important to note that fasting during cancer treatment is a complex approach that should be carefully evaluated and monitored by healthcare professionals. Cancer patients often experience various side effects from both the disease and the treatment, such as fatigue, nausea, and weight loss. Subjecting the body to prolonged fasting while undergoing radiation therapy can potentially accentuate these side effects and may not be advisable for all patients.

Additionally, the impact of fasting on each individual patient may vary depending on factors such as overall health, cancer type, stage, and treatment plan. Some patients may already experience unintentional weight loss or malnutrition due to the cancer itself, which can worsen with fasting. Therefore, a personalised approach considering the patient's specific circumstances is crucial when considering the integration of fasting with radiation therapy.

In conclusion, fasting has shown promise in improving the effectiveness of radiation therapy in cancer treatment through various mechanisms. However, it is essential for cancer patients to discuss this approach with their healthcare team before implementing it. Healthcare professionals can assess the patient's overall health, nutritional status, and treatment plan to determine if fasting could be a beneficial addition to their treatment regimen. Collaboration between patients and their healthcare providers is vital to ensure a safe and optimised treatment approach.

Fasting and Chemotherapy

Fasting and chemotherapy are two distinct approaches in the treatment of cancer patients that have been gaining attention in recent years. While chemotherapy aims to target and destroy cancer cells directly, fasting involves the voluntary abstinence from food for a specified period of time.

Fasting, particularly intermittent fasting or prolonged fasting, has been shown to have potential benefits for cancer patients undergoing chemotherapy. Several studies have suggested that fasting can help improve the efficacy of chemotherapy drugs while minimising the side effects.

One of the proposed mechanisms behind the potential synergy between fasting and chemotherapy is that fasting induces a state of metabolic stress in normal cells, making them more resistant to the toxic effects of chemotherapy. Meanwhile, cancer cells, which often have dysfunctional metabolic pathways, are more vulnerable to the effects of both chemotherapy and fasting.

Additionally, fasting has been shown to reduce levels of insulin-like growth factor 1 (IGF-1), a hormone that promotes cancer cell growth. Lower levels of IGF-1 may potentially inhibit the growth and spread of cancer cells, thereby enhancing the effectiveness of chemotherapy.

Moreover, fasting has shown promise in reducing the side effects associated with chemotherapy. Common side effects of chemotherapy include nausea, fatigue, and decreased immune function. Studies have indicated that fasting prior to chemotherapy treatments can help alleviate these side effects, improving the overall well-being and quality of life for cancer patients.

It is important to note that fasting should always be done under medical supervision, especially for cancer patients undergoing chemotherapy. Each patient's specific condition and treatment plan must be taken into consideration when implementing any dietary changes.

While research on the combination of fasting and chemotherapy is still emerging, the existing evidence suggests that fasting may be a complementary therapeutic strategy to enhance the effectiveness of chemotherapy and mitigate its side effects. However, further studies are needed to establish clear guidelines and protocols for implementing fasting in cancer treatment.

In conclusion, fasting, when done under medical supervision, may be a beneficial adjunct to chemotherapy for cancer patients. Its potential to enhance the efficacy of chemotherapy drugs while reducing side effects makes it an area of ongoing research and exploration. Ultimately, the decision to incorporate fasting into a cancer treatment plan should be made in consultation with healthcare professionals to ensure the safety and effectiveness for each individual patient.

Fasting and Immunotherapy

This is a Potential Combination for Cancer Patients

Cancer, a complex and devastating disease, affects millions of people worldwide. Over the years, various treatment strategies have been employed to combat cancer, ranging from surgery and radiation therapy to chemotherapy. However, emerging research suggests that the combination of fasting and immunotherapy may hold great promise for cancer patients.

Fasting, a practice that involves abstaining from food for a specific period, has been observed to have numerous health benefits. Apart from promoting weight loss and improving metabolic health, fasting has been shown to have a positive impact on the immune system. When an individual fasts, the body enters a state called ketosis, where it breaks down fat for energy instead of relying on glucose. This metabolic shift has been found to rejuvenate immune cells and enhance their functionality.

Immunotherapy, on the other hand, is a groundbreaking approach to cancer treatment that utilises the body's own immune system to target and destroy cancer cells. Unlike traditional treatments, such as chemotherapy, immunotherapy aims to boost the immune response against cancer while minimising damage to healthy cells. It has shown remarkable success in treating various types of cancers, including melanoma, lung cancer, and lymphoma.

Recently, researchers have turned their attention towards the potential synergy between fasting and immunotherapy. A study published in the journal Science Translational Medicine demonstrated that fasting prior to immunotherapy could significantly enhance the treatment's effectiveness. In mouse models, fasting led to an increased influx of immune cells into tumours and improved antitumor activity. These findings were attributed to the fact that fasting stimulates the release of certain immune cells from the bone marrow and reduces the levels of an immunosuppressive molecule called insulin-like growth factor-1 (IGF-1).

Furthermore, fasting was found to reduce the levels of glucose and certain amino acids in the blood, which are known to promote tumour growth. By starving tumour cells of these essential nutrients, fasting may make them more susceptible to the immune response triggered by immunotherapy. This combination approach has the potential to enhance tumour regression, prolong overall survival, and decrease the risk of cancer relapse.

While the results from animal studies are promising, it is important to note that these findings are preliminary, and more research is needed to validate the potential benefits of fasting in combination with immunotherapy for cancer patients. Clinical trials are underway to assess the safety and efficacy of this approach in human subjects.

It is also crucial to emphasise that fasting should be undertaken with caution and under the supervision of a healthcare professional, particularly for cancer patients who may already have compromised nutritional status. Fasting should never replace standard cancer treatments but should be considered as a supportive therapy or adjunct to existing treatments.

In conclusion, the combination of fasting and immunotherapy represents an intriguing approach to combating cancer. By leveraging the immune-boosting benefits of fasting alongside the targeted tumour-fighting capabilities of immunotherapy, researchers and healthcare professionals may be able to enhance treatment outcomes for cancer patients. Although further investigation is needed, this promising area of research offers hope for the future of cancer therapy.

Fasting and Surgery

Fasting is a topic of interest that has gained attention in recent years for its potential health benefits, including its impact on cancer patients undergoing surgery. While the concept may seem counterintuitive, research has shown that fasting before surgery may have various positive effects on cancer patients.

One significant benefit of fasting before surgery is that it can help improve the body's response to anaesthesia and reduce surgical complications. When a cancer patient fasts, their body enters a state of ketosis, where it starts using stored fats as an energy source instead of glucose. This metabolic shift can enhance the body's response to stress and decrease inflammation, which can ultimately minimise the risk of surgical complications.

Fasting has also been found to potentially reduce the side effects of chemotherapy and radiation therapy. These cancer treatments can cause side effects such as nausea, vomiting, and gastrointestinal issues. By fasting prior to surgery, patients may experience a decrease in these side effects due to the metabolic changes that occur during the fasting period.

Furthermore, fasting has been shown to have a positive impact on blood sugar levels. Cancer patients often experience changes in their blood sugar due to the disease itself or as a result of certain cancer treatments. By fasting, patients may be able to stabilise their blood sugar levels, which can be crucial for optimal surgical outcomes.

It is important to note that fasting before surgery should be carefully supervised and discussed with a healthcare professional, as the duration and type of fasting may vary depending on individual circumstances. The timing and duration of the fasting period may differ depending on the type of cancer, stage of the disease, and the specific surgical procedure being performed.

It is also crucial to consider that fasting alone should not be seen as a replacement for traditional cancer treatments. While there may be potential benefits, cancer patients should always consult their healthcare team and follow the recommended treatment plan established for their specific case.

In conclusion, fasting before surgery for cancer patients has shown promising benefits in terms of improving the body's response to anaesthesia, reducing surgical complications, managing side effects of cancer treatments, and stabilising blood sugar levels. However, it is essential to remember that fasting should always be done under the guidance of healthcare professionals, and it should not replace standard cancer treatments.

CHAPTER FIVE

Potential Challenges and Risks of Fasting for Cancer Patients

Impact of Fasting on Nutritional Status

Fasting has gained significant attention as a potential therapeutic strategy for cancer patients. It is believed that fasting can enhance the efficacy of cancer treatments and reduce the side effects associated with them. However, fasting also poses challenges and risks to the nutritional status of cancer patients, which must be carefully considered.

One of the primary challenges of fasting for cancer patients is the potential for nutrient deficiencies. Cancer patients already have increased nutritional needs due to the metabolic demands of the disease and the side effects of treatments. Fasting, especially prolonged or severe fasting, can further limit the intake of essential nutrients such as proteins, carbohydrates, fats, vitamins, and minerals. This can lead to malnutrition, impaired immune function, muscle wasting, and slowed wound healing, all of which can negatively impact the overall health and well-being of cancer patients.

Another challenge of fasting is the potential for muscle loss. Fasting triggers the body to utilise stored energy, including glycogen and body fat. However, in the absence of dietary intake, the body may also break down muscle tissue to meet its energy needs. For cancer patients who are already at risk of muscle wasting due to the disease and its treatments, fasting can exacerbate this issue, leading to further weakness and fatigue.

Furthermore, fasting can have detrimental effects on blood sugar control in cancer patients, especially those who have diabetes or are receiving certain cancer treatments. Without regular carbohydrate intake, blood glucose levels can drop dangerously low, leading to hypoglycemia. This can cause symptoms such as dizziness, weakness, confusion, and in severe cases, loss of consciousness. Additionally, fasting can make it difficult to manage diabetes medications or insulin levels, further exacerbating the risk of blood sugar imbalances.

Lastly, fasting can impact the mental and emotional well-being of cancer patients. Food is often associated with comfort, pleasure, and social interactions. Fasting for extended periods can lead to feelings of deprivation, isolation, and frustration, which can contribute to psychological distress and impact a patient's overall quality of life.

In conclusion, while fasting may hold potential benefits for cancer patients, it also presents challenges and risks to their nutritional status. Health care providers should carefully evaluate each patient's individual circumstances, including disease stage, treatment plan, nutritional needs, and overall health, before recommending or allowing fasting. Strategies to mitigate the potential risks, such as personalised fasting regimens and close monitoring of nutritional status, should be employed to ensure the well-being of cancer patients undergoing fasting as a part of their treatment plan.

Side Effects and Tolerance of Fasting

Fasting is the practice of abstaining from food or calorie intake for a certain period of time, and it has gained popularity as a means to improve health and potentially alleviate the side effects of various diseases, including cancer. However, while fasting might have benefits for some individuals, it also carries potential challenges and risks, especially for cancer patients. Two important aspects to consider in relation to fasting for cancer patients are the side effects and tolerance.

One challenge associated with fasting for cancer patients is the potential for increased side effects. Cancer treatments, such as chemotherapy or radiation therapy, often cause adverse effects like nausea, vomiting, and fatigue. These side effects can already be debilitating for patients, and fasting might exacerbate them. Without sufficient nutrients, the body may struggle to cope with the additional stress, potentially worsening the patient's overall well-being and quality of life.

Moreover, fasting can lead to nutrient deficiencies, which can have negative consequences for cancer patients. During fasting, the body lacks essential macronutrients (carbohydrates, proteins, and fats) as well as micronutrients (vitamins and minerals) necessary for proper functioning of the body's immune system and organ health. Cancer patients require adequate nutrition to support their immune system and aid in the recovery process. Therefore, fasting may compromise the patient's ability to fight off infections, decrease treatment effectiveness, and impede the body's ability to heal.

Another challenge of fasting for cancer patients is developing tolerance. Tolerance refers to the body's ability to endure fasting and the subsequent potential adaptation to the regimen. While some individuals may tolerate fasting well, cancer patients often have weakened immune systems and altered metabolism due to the disease and its treatments. The body's ability to adapt to fasting and its associated physiological changes may be compromised, leading to further physiological stress and potentially worsening the patient's condition.

Additionally, fasting can impact a cancer patient's emotional and psychological well-being. The restriction of food intake might cause feelings of deprivation, frustration, and anxiety, particularly for individuals undergoing cancer treatment already experiencing emotional distress. The mental and emotional toll of fasting can be counterproductive to the patient's overall mental health and may hinder their ability to cope with the challenges inherent in a cancer diagnosis.

In conclusion, while fasting has gained attention as a potential therapeutic approach for cancer patients, it is crucial to consider the challenges and risks associated with it. The side effects of cancer treatments, the potential for nutrient deficiencies, the difficulty in developing tolerance, and the impact on emotional well-being are crucial aspects to be mindful of when considering fasting for cancer patients. It is imperative for cancer patients to consult with their healthcare team before adopting any fasting regimen to ensure it is safe and appropriate for their unique circumstances.

Psychological and Emotional Challenges of Fasting

Fasting can be a challenging experience for anyone, but it can pose unique psychological and emotional challenges for cancer patients. Here are some of the issues that cancer patients might face when fasting:

1. Fear and Anxiety:

Cancer patients may already be dealing with a wide range of fears and anxieties related to their diagnosis and treatment. Fasting can amplify these feelings as they worry about how to manage their nutrition and maintain their strength during the fasting period. This fear can also stem from concerns about whether fasting will negatively impact their treatment outcomes.

2. Coping with Loss of Control:

Fasting is a voluntary act of abstaining from food, but cancer patients may feel a loss of control over their bodies when they already have to relinquish control to medical professionals for their treatment. This loss of control can further enhance feelings of vulnerability and helplessness.

3. Emotional Turmoil:

Cancer patients often experience a rollercoaster of emotions, including anger, sadness, and fear. Fasting can add another layer of emotional turmoil as the body adjusts to the changes in routine and sustenance. Hunger pangs and physical discomfort can worsen mood swings and emotional instability.

4. Social Isolation:

Fasting typically involves abstaining from food and sometimes even refraining from social activities centred around meals. This can lead to feelings of

isolation and exclusion from social gatherings,
which may be particularly distressing for cancer
patients who may already feel isolated due to their
illness.

5. Body Image Concerns:

Cancer treatments can cause significant changes in
a person's physical appearance, such as hair loss,
weight gain or loss, and changes in skin texture.
Fasting may further impact body image concerns
for cancer patients, especially if it results in
additional weight loss or changes in their physical
appearance.

6. Guilt and Shame:

Cancer patients may experience guilt or shame if
they are unable to adhere to fasting rituals or
dietary restrictions due to their medical condition or
treatment side effects. They may feel as though
they are failing or not doing enough to improve their
health.

It is important for cancer patients who choose to
fast to have strong emotional support from
healthcare professionals, family, and friends.
Engaging in open and honest communication with
their healthcare team about fasting plans can help
address potential concerns and provide guidance
on how to manage any psychological or emotional
challenges that may arise. Additionally, seeking
professional counselling or joining support groups

can provide a safe space for patients to express
their emotions and receive the necessary support
during this challenging time.

CHAPTER SIX

Integrating Fasting into Cancer Care: Practical Considerations

Collaborating with Healthcare Professionals

Collaboration is a crucial aspect of providing comprehensive and effective cancer care. In-depth collaboration with healthcare professionals from various disciplines ensures that patients receive the best possible treatment and support throughout their cancer journey. By working together, medical oncologists, surgeons, radiation oncologists, nurses, pharmacists, and other specialists can combine their expertise and resources to develop personalised and multidisciplinary treatment plans.

One key benefit of collaborating with healthcare professionals is the ability to gather diverse perspectives and knowledge. Cancer care involves a complex array of treatments, including surgery, chemotherapy, radiation therapy, immunotherapy, and targeted therapies. Each of these treatments has its own unique considerations and potential side effects. By collaborating, healthcare professionals can collectively discuss and evaluate different treatment options, considering factors such as the stage and type of cancer, the patient's overall health, and the desired outcome. This collaborative approach ensures that all possible treatment avenues are explored and that patients receive the most appropriate and effective therapies.

In addition to treatment planning, collaboration is vital in aspects of support and survivorship. Social workers, psychologists, and palliative care specialists can play a crucial role in addressing the emotional and psychological needs of cancer patients and their families. By working together, healthcare professionals can ensure that patients have access to the necessary social, psychological, and spiritual support services throughout their cancer journey.

Collaboration also extends to research and clinical trials, which drive advancements in cancer treatment and improve patient outcomes. Many breakthroughs in cancer care have been the result of collaborative research efforts among scientists, clinicians, and pharmaceutical companies. By partnering with healthcare professionals across different institutions and organisations, researchers can share knowledge, resources, and expertise, accelerating the development of new therapies and treatment approaches.

Furthermore, collaboration with healthcare professionals promotes continuity of care for cancer patients. As treatment progresses, it is crucial for various healthcare providers to communicate and coordinate their efforts to provide consistent monitoring, follow-up, and post-treatment care. Effective collaboration ensures that critical information is shared and that any potential complications or side effects are addressed promptly.

However, effective collaboration requires clear communication, mutual respect, and shared decision-making among healthcare professionals. Regular interdisciplinary team meetings, tumour boards, and case conferences can facilitate open discussions and promote consensus-driven decision-making, leading to a more comprehensive and personalised approach to cancer care.

In conclusion, collaboration with healthcare professionals is essential for providing optimal and comprehensive cancer care. By working together, healthcare professionals can combine their expertise, resources, and perspectives to develop personalised treatment plans, address the emotional and psychological needs of patients, advance research efforts, and ensure continuity of care. Through effective collaboration, healthcare professionals can make a significant difference in the lives of cancer patients and contribute to improved patient outcomes.

Monitoring and Assessing Progress during Fasting

Monitoring and assessing progress during fasting is crucial to ensure the safety and effectiveness of the fasting regimen. Fasting refers to the voluntary abstention from food and, in some cases, fluids for a specified period. It has gained interest in cancer care due to its potential benefits, such as enhancing the efficacy of chemotherapy, reducing side effects, and improving quality of life.

To monitor and assess progress during fasting for cancer care, several factors need to be considered:

1. Medical Evaluation: Before starting a fasting regimen, it is essential to conduct a thorough medical evaluation to assess the patient's overall health and suitability for fasting. Blood tests, imaging scans, and consultations with other specialists may be part of this evaluation.

2. Nutritional Assessment: Adequate nutrition is crucial for cancer patients to maintain strength and support their immune system. It is essential to assess the patient's nutritional status before fasting and ensure they receive adequate calories, macronutrients, and micronutrients during the fasting period. Regular monitoring of weight, body composition, and nutritional markers can help identify any deficiencies or imbalances.

3. Regular Medical Check-ups: Regular medical check-ups are necessary to monitor the patient's health during fasting. These check-ups may include physical examinations, blood tests, and imaging studies to assess any changes in the disease status or potential side effects of fasting.

4. Monitoring for Side Effects: Fasting can lead to side effects such as fatigue, dizziness, electrolyte imbalances, and dehydration. Close monitoring of vital signs, fluid intake, urine output, and symptoms such as nausea, vomiting, or weakness is essential to identify and manage any adverse effects promptly.

5. Follow-up Imaging and Biomarkers: Depending on the cancer type and stage, imaging studies such as CT scans, PET scans, or tumour markers may be used to assess the response to fasting and treatment. These tests can help determine if the fasting regimen is having a positive impact on the disease progression.

6. Quality of Life Assessment: Assessing the patient's quality of life is crucial during fasting for cancer care. Validated questionnaires or surveys can be used to measure physical, emotional, and social well-being. Regular assessment of quality of life can help determine if fasting is improving or detrimentally affecting the patient's overall well-being.

7. Multidisciplinary Collaboration: Monitoring and assessing progress during fasting for cancer care should involve a multidisciplinary team of healthcare professionals, including oncologists, nutritionists, dietitians, and supportive care specialists. The team can collaboratively evaluate the patient's progress, adjust the fasting regimen or supportive measures as needed, and address any concerns or complications that may arise.

In conclusion, monitoring and assessing progress during fasting for cancer care is crucial to ensure the safety and effectiveness of the fasting regimen. Regular medical evaluations, nutritional assessments, monitoring for side effects, follow-up imaging and biomarkers, and quality of life assessments are essential components of the monitoring process. By closely monitoring the patient's health and well-being, healthcare professionals can tailor the fasting regimen to optimise outcomes and provide the best possible care for cancer patients.

Developing Individualised Fasting Plans

Developing individualised fasting plans for cancer care is an emerging and promising area of research that aims to enhance the effectiveness of cancer treatment and improve overall patient outcomes. Fasting, or the deliberate restriction of caloric intake for a specified period, has been shown to have various effects on the body that may influence cancer progression and treatment response. However, it is crucial to note that individualised fasting plans should be developed in collaboration with healthcare professionals, considering the specific needs and medical history of each patient.

Understanding the Basis of Fasting in Cancer Care:

1. Metabolic Alterations:
Fasting induces metabolic changes in the body, such as a shift from glucose to ketone metabolism. Cancer cells often rely heavily on glucose for energy, and fasting may create an environment that is less favourable for their growth.

2. Autophagy Activation:
Fasting triggers autophagy, a cellular process that removes damaged components and promotes cellular recycling. This can be particularly relevant in cancer treatment, as it may help eliminate dysfunctional cells.

3. Enhanced Treatment Tolerance:
Fasting has been shown to enhance the tolerability of certain cancer treatments, such as chemotherapy. By protecting normal cells from the toxic effects of treatment, fasting may allow for higher doses to be administered, potentially improving therapeutic outcomes.

1. Patient Assessment:

Conduct a thorough assessment of the patient's medical history, current health status, type of cancer, and any ongoing cancer treatments. This information is critical for tailoring a fasting plan that is safe and effective for the individual.

2. Duration and Type of Fasting:

Determine the appropriate duration and type of fasting for the patient. Options include intermittent fasting, extended fasting, or periodic fasting mimicking diets. The choice depends on factors such as the cancer type, stage, and the patient's ability to adhere to the plan.

3. Nutritional Support:

Ensure that patients receive proper nutritional support before, during, and after fasting periods. This may involve working with a registered dietitian to develop a plan that provides essential nutrients and maintains overall health.

4. Monitoring and Adaptation:

Regularly monitor the patient's response to the fasting plan. Adjustments may be necessary based on changes in the patient's health status, treatment regimen, or tolerance to fasting.

5. Patient Education and Support:

Educate patients about the rationale behind the fasting plan, potential benefits, and any associated risks. Provide support to help them adhere to the plan and address any concerns or challenges they may encounter.

It's essential to emphasise that developing individualised fasting plans for cancer care requires a collaborative approach involving oncologists, dietitians, and other healthcare professionals. The goal is to integrate fasting strategies as a complementary element to conventional cancer treatments, with the aim of improving treatment efficacy and the overall well-being of the patient.

In conclusion, the field of individualised fasting plans for cancer care holds promise, but it is crucial to approach it with caution and in consultation with healthcare professionals. Rigorous research, combined with personalised care, will contribute to the development of evidence-based strategies that can optimise cancer treatment outcomes.

Addressing Dietary and Nutritional Needs during Fasting

Addressing dietary and nutritional needs during fasting is crucial to ensure that individuals maintain their health and well-being while abstaining from food for a specified period. Fasting is a practice observed for various reasons, including religious, spiritual, or health purposes. Regardless of the motivation behind fasting, it's essential to approach it with careful consideration of one's nutritional requirements. Here are some key considerations and tips for addressing dietary and nutritional needs during fasting:

1. Pre-Fasting Preparation:
   - Before starting a fast, it's important to ensure that the individual is in good health and has no underlying nutritional deficiencies. A balanced and nutritious diet leading up to the fast can help build reserves of essential nutrients.

2. Hydration:
   - Staying hydrated is crucial during fasting. Water consumption should be sufficient to prevent dehydration. Herbal teas and infusions are also good options. However, beverages containing caffeine or excessive sugar should be limited.

3. Suhoor/Sehri (Pre-dawn Meal):
   - The pre-dawn meal is crucial as it provides the energy needed for the day. To offer sustained energy, include complex carbohydrates, protein, and healthy fats. Whole grains, eggs, yoghurt, fruits, and nuts are good choices.

4. Iftar (Breaking the Fast):
   - Break the fast with a combination of hydrating foods and those that provide quick energy. Dates and water are commonly used to break the fast,

followed by a balanced meal. Include foods from many food groups, such as lean proteins, whole grains, veggies, and fruits.

5. Balanced Nutrition:
- Ensure that each meal includes a balance of macronutrients (carbohydrates, proteins, and fats) and micronutrients (vitamins and minerals). This helps in meeting overall nutritional needs.

6. Avoid Overeating:
- While breaking the fast, it's important not to overeat. Eating slowly and mindfully can help prevent digestive discomfort. Small, nutrient-dense meals are preferable.

7. Foods to Prioritise:
- Emphasise nutrient-dense foods like fruits, vegetables, whole grains, lean proteins, and healthy fats. These foods provide essential vitamins, minerals, and antioxidants.

8. Supplementation:
- Depending on the length and type of fast, supplementation may be necessary. Consult with a healthcare professional to determine if additional vitamins or minerals are needed.

9. Monitor Blood Sugar Levels:
- Individuals with diabetes or other metabolic conditions should carefully monitor their blood sugar levels during fasting. It may be necessary to

adjust medication or consult a healthcare
professional for guidance.

10. Listen to the Body:
   - Be aware of hunger and satiety cues. It's
essential to be attuned to the body's signals and
adjust the fasting routine if needed.

11. Post-Fasting Rehydration:
   - After the fast, rehydrate with water and
electrolyte-rich beverages to replenish fluids lost
during the fasting period.

12. Consult with Professionals:
   - Individuals with specific health conditions or
those on medication should consult with healthcare
professionals or registered dietitians before starting
a fast.

In conclusion, addressing dietary and nutritional
needs during fasting requires a thoughtful and
well-planned approach. By incorporating a variety
of nutrient-dense foods, staying hydrated, and
considering individual health conditions, individuals
can observe fasting periods while maintaining their
overall health and well-being.

CHAPTER SEVEN

Future Directions and Research Opportunities

Current Research on Fasting and Cancer

In recent years, there has been growing interest among scientists and researchers in studying the effects of fasting on cancer. Fasting, which involves voluntarily abstaining from eating or reducing calorie intake for a specific period of time, has been shown to have potential benefits in cancer prevention and treatment.

One area of research focuses on how fasting can affect cancer growth and progression. Studies conducted on both animal models and human subjects have shown that fasting can inhibit the growth of tumours and increase the effectiveness of cancer treatments such as chemotherapy. Fasting triggers metabolic changes in the body, including a decrease in insulin levels and an increase in ketone bodies, which have been associated with inhibiting cancer cell growth. It is believed that cancer cells are less able to adapt to these metabolic changes and, therefore, can be more vulnerable to treatment during fasting.

Furthermore, fasting has been found to enhance the immune system's ability to target and destroy cancer cells. Researchers have observed that fasting can promote autophagy, a cellular process in which damaged or dysfunctional components are recycled or eliminated. This process helps to regenerate healthy cells and remove potentially harmful ones, including cancer cells. Additionally, fasting has been shown to reduce the production of certain growth factors that promote tumour growth and metastasis, thereby potentially limiting the spread of cancer.

Another area of interest in fasting and cancer research is its potential for reducing the side effects of cancer treatments. Several studies have suggested that fasting prior to or during chemotherapy can protect healthy cells from the toxic effects of treatment. Fasting has been shown to induce protective mechanisms in normal cells, making them more resistant to chemotherapy-induced damage. This can potentially minimise the side effects of chemotherapy, such as nausea, hair loss, and reduced immune function.

Despite these promising findings, it is important to note that the field of fasting and cancer research is still relatively new, and further investigations are needed to fully understand its mechanisms of action and potential applications. Clinical trials involving larger sample sizes, diverse cancer types, and long-term follow-ups are necessary to determine the optimal fasting protocols and identify any potential risks associated with this approach.

In conclusion, current research on fasting and cancer suggests that it may have significant benefits in cancer prevention, treatment, and minimising chemotherapy-associated side effects. While more studies are warranted, these findings provide a promising foundation for future research and potential integration of fasting as an adjunct therapy for cancer.

Promising Areas for Further Exploration

1. Combination therapies:

Further exploration can be done on combining fasting with other treatment modalities, such as chemotherapy or immunotherapy. It would be interesting to investigate whether fasting can enhance the effectiveness of these therapies by sensitising cancer cells or making them more susceptible to treatment.

2. Fasting mimicking diets:

While traditional fasting has shown promising results, there is growing interest in studying the effects of fasting mimicking diets (FMDs) on cancer. FMDs involve calorie restriction or specific dietary modifications that mimic the effects of fasting. More research can be conducted to determine the optimal duration and composition of FMDs for cancer treatment.

3. Fasting as an adjunct therapy:

Investigating the potential of fasting as an adjunct therapy alongside conventional cancer treatments is another area for exploration. Studies could focus on the effects of fasting on treatment side effects, such as reducing toxicity and improving quality of life for cancer patients.

4. Role of fasting in cancer prevention:

While much of the current research focuses on fasting as a treatment for cancer, further exploration can be done on its role in cancer prevention. Understanding whether fasting can lower the risk of cancer development and recurrence could have significant implications for public health.

5. Mechanisms of action:

Although there is some understanding of how fasting affects cancer cells, further research is needed to elucidate the underlying mechanisms. Studying the molecular and cellular changes that occur during fasting can provide valuable insights into the pathways involved and help identify potential targets for therapeutic intervention.

6. Personalised fasting strategies:

Investigating the concept of personalised fasting strategies for cancer patients can be an interesting avenue to explore. Understanding how factors such as patient-specific characteristics, tumour type, and stage influence the response to fasting can help tailor fasting protocols to individual patients for maximum efficacy.

7. Long-term effects and safety:

While fasting has shown promise in preclinical and early clinical studies, more research is needed to evaluate the long-term effects and safety of fasting in cancer patients. Studies focusing on the potential risks, such as malnutrition or muscle loss, associated with prolonged fasting can help guide the development of safe and effective fasting protocols.

Overall, further exploration of these areas can provide valuable insights into the potential benefits and limitations of fasting as a therapeutic approach in cancer treatment and prevention.

Potential Integration into Cancer Treatment Guidelines

Cancer treatment guidelines, also known as clinical practice guidelines, are evidence-based recommendations that help healthcare professionals make informed decisions about the best approaches to diagnosing and treating cancer. These guidelines serve as a valuable resource for clinicians and researchers, ensuring standardisation and consistency in the delivery of care.

Integrating new potential treatments into cancer treatment guidelines is a crucial step in advancing patient care and optimising treatment outcomes. With the rapid progress in biomedical research and the development of novel therapies, it is imperative to regularly review and update these guidelines to incorporate the latest scientific evidence.

Here are some key considerations for the potential integration of new therapies into cancer treatment guidelines:

1. Robust clinical trial evidence: Integration into treatment guidelines typically requires substantial evidence from well-designed clinical trials. The results should demonstrate clear benefits, compared to standard treatment options, in terms of survival rates, disease-free intervals, quality of life, or other relevant endpoints.

2. Comparative effectiveness: Incorporating new therapies into guidelines necessitates a comparison with existing treatments. Assessing the relative efficacy, safety, and cost-effectiveness of the new intervention against established standards is crucial to guide treatment decisions.

3. Patient-centred outcomes: Guidelines should prioritise patient-centred outcomes, considering factors such as quality of life, functional status, symptom control, and treatment-related toxicities. Integration of new therapies should carefully evaluate the impact on patients' overall well-being and their ability to maintain normal daily activities.

4. Multidisciplinary approach: Cancer treatment often involves a multidisciplinary team comprising medical oncologists, surgeons, radiation oncologists, and other healthcare professionals. The integration process should engage experts from various disciplines to ensure comprehensive and well-rounded clinical recommendations.

5. Regular guideline updates: Given the rapid pace of advancements in cancer research, treatment guidelines should be regularly updated to reflect the evolving scientific landscape. A periodic review process is essential to incorporate new evidence and therapeutic options promptly.

6. Consideration of accessibility and affordability: As new therapies often come with higher costs, guidelines should also account for their accessibility and affordability. Balancing the benefits and costs is crucial to ensure equity in access to effective treatments for all cancer patients.

7. Real-world evidence: Clinical trials provide vital initial evidence, but real-world data can further validate the effectiveness and safety of new therapies. Incorporating real-world evidence, such as data from patient registries or post-marketing surveillance, can enhance the confidence around integrating novel treatments into guidelines.

In conclusion, integrating new potential therapies into cancer treatment guidelines plays a crucial role in optimising patient care and improving outcomes. By critically evaluating clinical trial evidence, considering patient-centred outcomes, and embracing a multidisciplinary approach, guidelines can effectively incorporate new therapies and ensure the highest standard of care for cancer patients. Regular updates and the consideration of accessibility and affordability further enhance the relevance and practicality of these guidelines.

CONCLUSION

Fasting as a Complementary Approach to Cancer Care

Fasting, the voluntary abstinence from food and sometimes drink for a specified period, has been practised for centuries for various reasons. In recent years, fasting has gained attention as a potential complementary approach to cancer care. While it is essential to note that fasting cannot replace conventional cancer treatments such as chemotherapy or radiation therapy, emerging research suggests that it may offer some benefits when used alongside traditional treatments.

One of the primary mechanisms behind the potential benefits of fasting in cancer care is its ability to induce a state of cellular stress called "metabolic stress." This stress condition triggers a series of metabolic changes in the body that can potentially enhance the effectiveness of cancer treatment. During fasting, the body switches its energy source from glucose to ketones, which are produced from fat stores. This metabolic switch not only weakens cancer cells that primarily rely on glucose for growth but also activates various cellular defence mechanisms.

Several animal studies have shown that fasting can enhance the effectiveness and reduce the side effects of chemotherapy. Animal models have demonstrated that fasting prior to chemotherapy treatments can selectively protect healthy cells while making cancer cells more susceptible to the effects of chemotherapy drugs. As a result, fasting may help increase the efficacy of chemotherapy, allowing for lower drug doses and potentially fewer side effects.

Fasting has also shown promise in improving the body's immune response to cancer. Animal studies have revealed that fasting can lead to a rejuvenation of the immune system, with an increase in the production of new immune cells and improved immune function. A strong immune system is essential in fighting cancer as it helps identify and destroy malignant cells. By boosting the immune system, fasting may indirectly aid in the body's ability to combat cancer.

Furthermore, fasting has been found to reduce inflammation, a key factor in tumour growth and progression. Chronic inflammation can generate an environment that encourages cancer cell survival and multiplication. By reducing inflammation, fasting may inhibit the growth and spread of cancer, as well as alleviate cancer-related symptoms.

It is important to highlight that fasting should always be approached with caution, especially for cancer patients. Each individual's circumstance is unique, and consulting with a healthcare professional is crucial before considering any fasting regimen. Additionally, it is essential to implement proper hydration and nutritional support during fasting to mitigate potential risks.

In conclusion, fasting as a complementary approach to cancer care holds promise and is gaining attention in the medical field. Although more research is needed to understand its full potential, initial studies suggest that fasting, when used alongside conventional cancer treatments, may enhance their effectiveness, reduce side effects, boost immune function, and alleviate inflammation. As our understanding of fasting and its impact on cancer grows, it may become an integral part of an integrative cancer care approach, providing an additional tool to improve patient outcomes.

Recommendations for Patients, Healthcare Providers, and Researchers

Fasting, the intentional abstention from food for a specified period, has garnered attention in the context of cancer prevention and treatment. While preliminary research suggests potential benefits, it's crucial to approach fasting with caution and informed decision-making. Here are recommendations tailored for patients, healthcare providers, and researchers.

1. Consult with Your Healthcare Team:

- Before considering any fasting regimen, consult your oncologist or healthcare provider. They can assess your individual health status, treatment plan, and overall well-being to determine if fasting is safe and suitable for you.

2. Educate Yourself:

- Understand the different fasting methods, such as intermittent fasting, prolonged fasting, or time-restricted eating. Be aware of potential side effects and how fasting may interact with your specific cancer type and treatment.

3. Timing Matters:

- If considering fasting during cancer treatment, choose the timing wisely. Avoid fasting on days when you receive chemotherapy or other intensive treatments. Your body needs adequate energy and nutrients during these times.

4. Stay Hydrated:

- Ensure proper hydration during fasting periods. Water is essential for maintaining overall health and supporting the body's natural detoxification processes.

5. Monitor Your Body:

- Pay close attention to the messages sent by your body. If you experience adverse effects, such as dizziness, weakness, or nausea, discontinue fasting and consult your healthcare team immediately.

1. Individualized Approach:
   - Recognize that each cancer patient is unique. Consider the patient's overall health, cancer type, stage, and ongoing treatments when evaluating the feasibility of fasting.

2. Collaborative Decision-Making:
   - Engage in open and honest communication with patients about the potential benefits and risks of fasting. Encourage them to share their intentions with you and make decisions collaboratively.

3. Continuous Monitoring:
   - Regularly monitor patients who choose to fast during cancer treatment. Assess their nutritional status, weight, and overall well-being. Adjust recommendations accordingly to ensure optimal support.

4. Educational Support:
   - Provide patients with reliable educational materials on fasting and cancer. Address common misconceptions and emphasize the importance of combining fasting, if deemed appropriate, with a balanced and nutrient-rich diet.

5. Research Collaboration:

- Encourage participation in clinical trials that investigate the impact of fasting on specific cancer types. Contribute to the growing body of evidence to refine guidelines and enhance patient care.

For Researchers

1. Diversify Study Populations:

- Ensure that research studies include diverse populations with various cancer types, stages, and demographic characteristics. This will contribute to a more comprehensive understanding of the potential effects of fasting.

2. Long-Term Impact Assessment:

- Design studies that assess the long-term impact of fasting on cancer survivors, considering factors such as recurrence rates, quality of life, and overall survival. This will provide a more comprehensive view of fasting's role in cancer care.

3. Mechanistic Studies:

- Investigate the underlying mechanisms through which fasting may influence cancer biology. Understanding the molecular and cellular processes can guide the development of targeted interventions and personalized treatment approaches.

4. Collaboration with Healthcare Providers:

- Foster collaboration between researchers and healthcare providers to bridge the gap between scientific knowledge and clinical practice. This will facilitate the translation of research findings into evidence-based guidelines.

5. Public Awareness:
- Engage in science communication to disseminate research findings responsibly. Emphasize the evolving nature of the field and the importance of evidence-based decision-making, discouraging unsupported or extreme fasting practices.

Conclusion:

Fasting and its potential impact on cancer treatment and prevention are areas of ongoing research. Patients, healthcare providers, and researchers play crucial roles in navigating this evolving landscape. By adopting an informed and collaborative approach, we can better understand the nuanced relationship between fasting and cancer and optimize patient outcomes.

DETOX

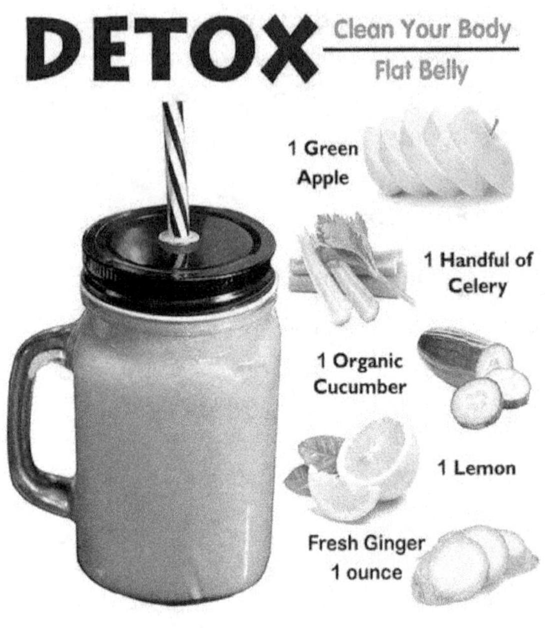

DETOX
Clean Your Body
Flat Belly
1 Green Apple
1 Handful of Celery
1 Organic Cucumber
1 Lemon
Fresh Ginger 1 ounce